NURSING
Crossword Puzzle For Student Nurses
Volume 1
Issue 3

MW01152989

PHARMACOLOGY

Evelyn Justiniano LPN, GRN

MEDICATION ANTIDOTES

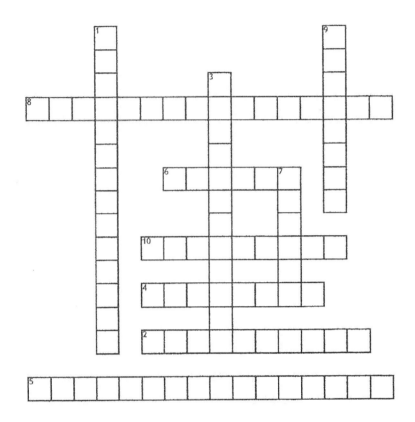

Across
2. What is Potassium's antidote?
4. What is digoxin antidote?
5. What is Magnesium Sulfate antidote?
6. What are Opiods antidote?
8. What is Heparin's antidote?
10. What is Benzodiazepines antidote?

Down
1. What is tylenol's antidote?
3. What is Iron's antidote?
7. What are Narcotics antidote?
9. What is Coumadin's antidote?

NON BENZODIAZEPINE, NONBARBITURATE CNS AGENTS FOR ANXIETY AND INSOMNIA

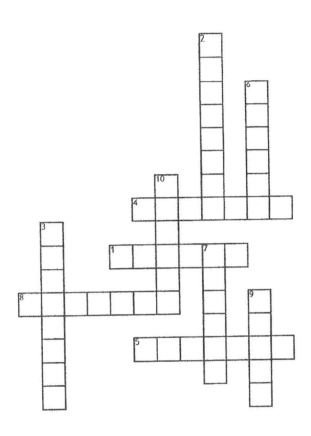

Across

1. What is Buspirone trade name?
4. What is Propranolol trade name?
5. What is Eszopiclone trade name?
8. What is Ramelteon trade name?

Down

2. What is Valproate trade name?
3. What is Atenolol trade name?
6. What is Zaleplon trade name?
7. What is Zolpidem trade name?
9. What s Diphenhydramine trade name?
10. What is Doxylamine trade name?

ATTENTION DEFICIT-HYPERACTIVITY DISORDER CNS STIMULANTS & NONSTIMULANTS MEDICATIONS

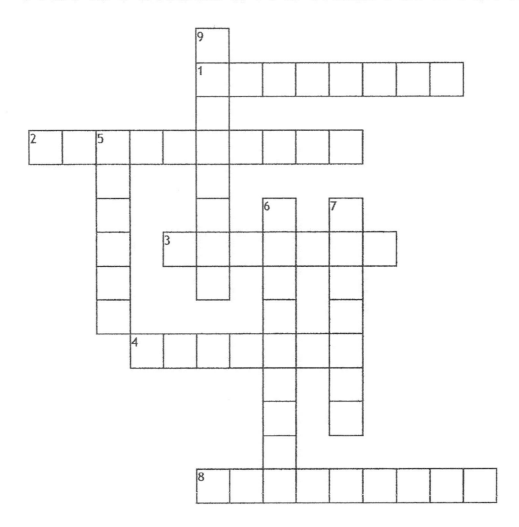

Across

1. What is d- & l-Amphetamine racemic mixture trade name?

2. What is Dextroamphetamine mixture trade name?

3. What is Methamphetamine trade name?

4. What is Methylphenidate trade name?

8. What is Atomoxetine trade name?

Down

5. What is Benzphetamine trade name?

6. What is Dexmethylphenidate trade name?

7. What is Lisdexamfetamine trade name?

9. What is Clonidine trade name?

SELECTIVE SEROTONIN REUPTAKE INHIBITORS (SSRIs) & SEROTONIN-NOREPINEPHRINE REUPTAKE INHIBITORS (SNRIs)

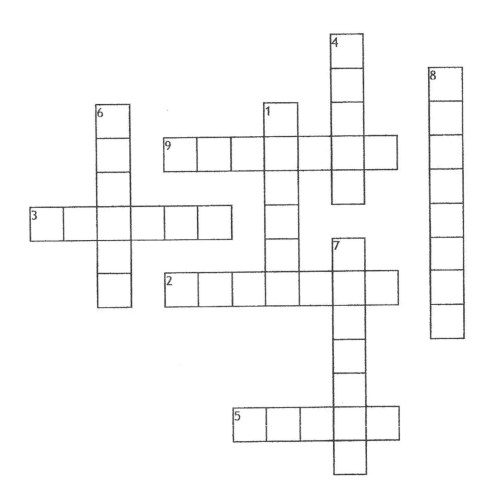

Across

2. What is Escitalopram Oxalate trade name?
3. What is Fluoxetine trade name?
5. What is Paroxetine trade name?
9. What is Venlafaxine trade name?

Down

1. What is Citalopram trade name?
4. What is Fluvoxamine trade name?
6. What is Sertraline trade name?
7. What is Desvenlafaxine trade name?
8. What is Duloxetine trade name?

ANTICONVULSANT MEDICATIONS

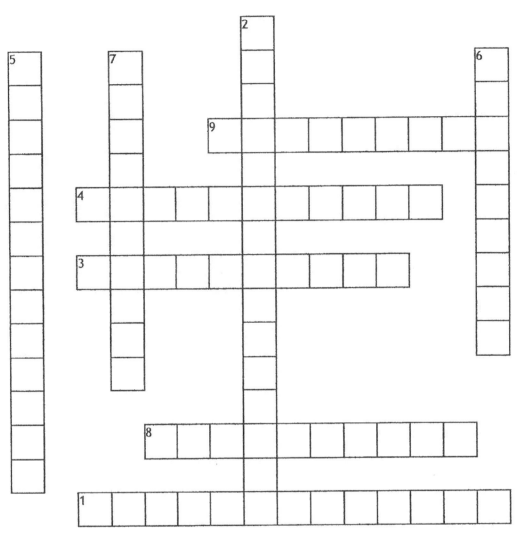

Across
1. What is Tegretol generic name?
3. What is Neurontin generic name?
4. What is Lamictal generic name?
8. What is Topamax generic name?
9. What is Depacon generic name?

Down
2. What is Depakote generic name?
5. What is luminal generic name?
6. What is Dilantin generic name?
7. What is Lyrica generic name?

ANTIPSYCHOTIC MEDICATIONS

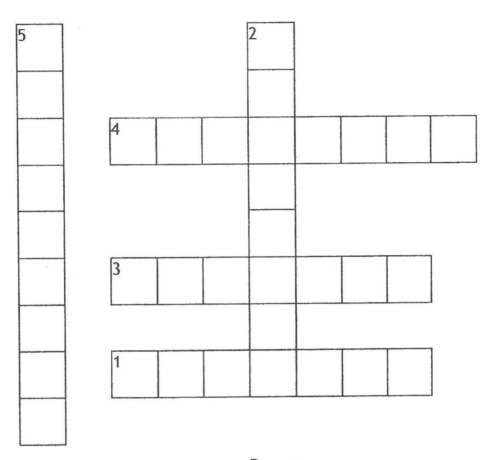

Across
1. What is Aripiprazole trade name?
3. What is Olanzepine trade name?
4. What is Quetiapine Fumarate trade name?

Down
2. What s Clozapine trade name?
5. What is Risperidone trade name?

PARKINSON'S ANTICHOLINERGIC MEDS

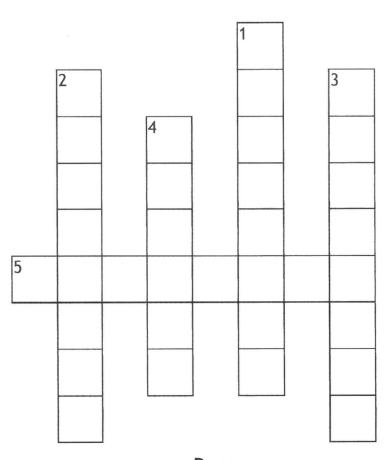

Across

5. What is Procyclidine trade name?

Down

1. What is Diphenhydramine trade name?
2. What is Biperiden trade name?
3. What is Benzotropine trade name?
4. What is Trihexyphenidyl trade name?

PARKINSON'S DOPAMINERGIC MEDICATIONS

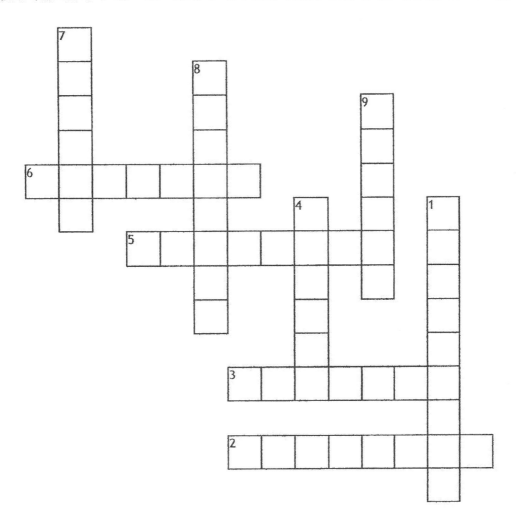

Across

2. What is Bromocriptine trade name?
3. What is Carbidopa-Levodopa trade name?
5. What is levadopa trade name?
6. What is Pramipexole trade name?

Down

1. What is Amantadine trade name?
4. What is Entacapone trade name?
7. What is Ropinirole trade name?
8. What is Selegiline trade name?
9. What is Tolcapone trade name?

ALZHEIMER'S ACETYLCHOLINESTERASE INHIBITORS MEDICATIONS

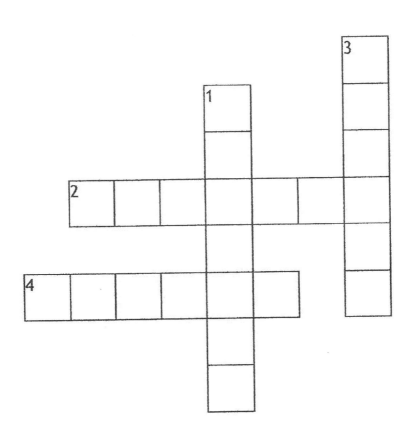

Across

2. What is Galantamine trade name?

4. What is Tacrine trade name?

Down

1. What is Donepezil trade name?

3. What is Rivastigmine Tartrate trade name?

MULTIPLE SCLEROSIS MEDICATIONS

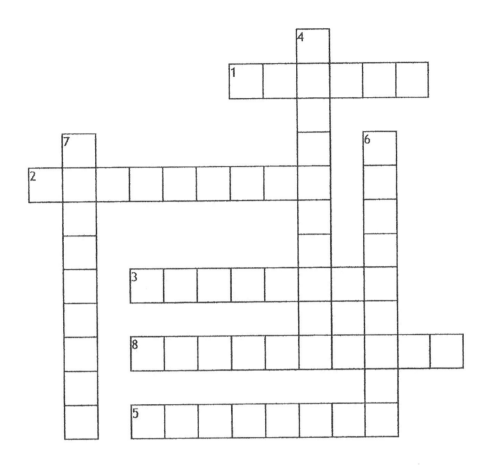

Across

1. What is Interferon beta-1 a trade name?
2. What is Interferon beta-1 b trade name?
3. What is Glatiramer Acetate trade name?
5. What is Modafinil trade name?
8. What is Methylprednisolone trade name?

Down

4. What is Mitoxantrone trade name?
6. What s Amantadine trade name?
7. What is Gabapentin trade name?

NONPHENOTHIAZINES CONVENTIONAL ANTIPSYCHOTICS MEDICATIONS

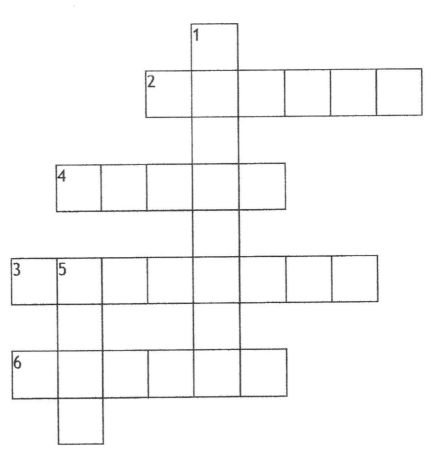

Across

2. What is Haloperidol trade name?

3. What is Loxapine Succinate trade name?

4. What is Molindone HCL trade name?

6. What is Thiothixene HCL trade name?

Down

1. What is Chlorprothixene trade name?

5. What is Pimozide trade name?

SYMPATHOMIMETICS MEDICATIONS

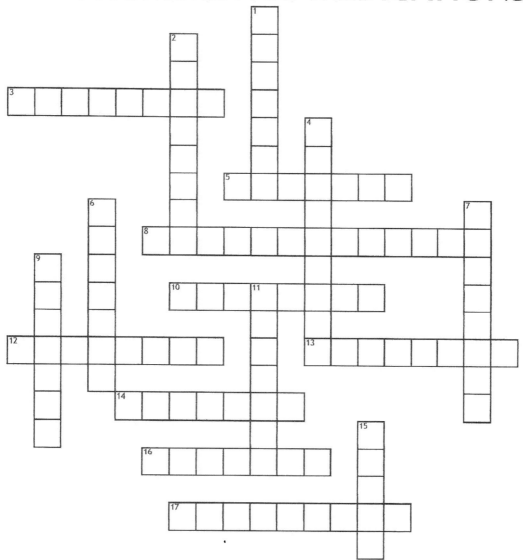

Across

3. What is Dexmedetomidine HCL trade name?
5. What is methyldopa trade name?
8. What is Phenylephrine trade name?
10. What is Dobutamine trade name?
12. What is Clonidine trade name?
13. What is norepinephrine trade name?
14. What is Formoterol trade name?
16. What is Metaproterenol trade name?
17. What is Ephinephrine trade name?

Down

1. What is Isoproterenol trade name?
2. What is Terbutaline trade name?
4. What is Albuterol trade name?
6. What is Ritodrine trade name?
7. What is Salmeterol trade name?
9. What is Pseudophedrine trade name?
11. What is Metaraminol trade name?
15. What is Oxymetazoline trade name?

PARASYMPATHOMIMETICS MEDICATIONS

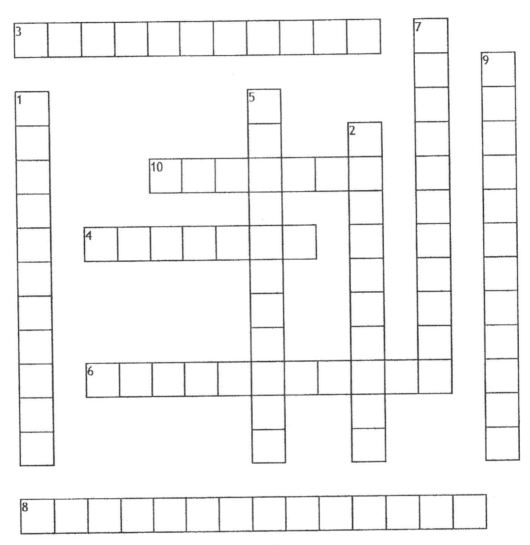

Across

3. What is Mytelase generic name?
4. What is Donepezil generic name?
6. What is Prostigmin generic name?
8. What is Mestinon generic name?
10. What is Cognex generic name?

Down

1. What is Urecholine generic name?
2. What is Evoxac generic name?
5. What is Tensilon generic name?
7. What is Isopto Carpine generic name?
9. What is Exelon generic name?

PARASYMPATHOMIMETIC MEDICATIONS II

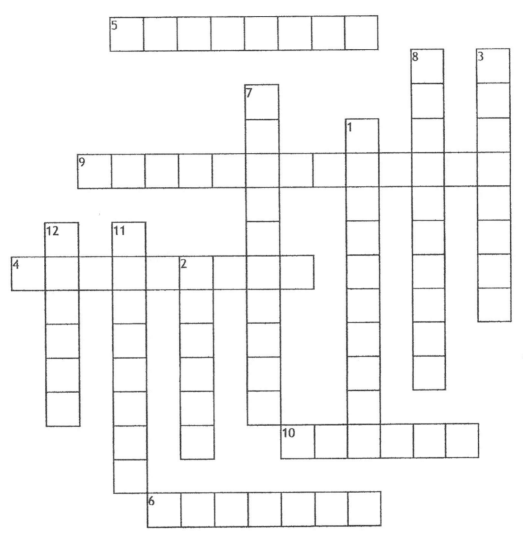

Across

4. What is the trade name for Aricept?
5. What is the trade name for Edrophonium?
6. What is the trade name for Galantamine Hydrobromide
9. What is the trade name for Pilocarpine?
10. What is the trade name for Rivastigmine?

Down

1. What is the trade name for Bethanechol?
2. What is the trade name for Cevimeline HCL
3. What is the trade name for Amebenonium CHL?
7. What is the trade name for Neostigmine?
8. What is the trade name for Physostigmine?
11. What is the trade name for Pyridostigmine?
12. What is the trade name for Tacrine?

NUEROMUSCULAR BLOCKING MEDICATIONS

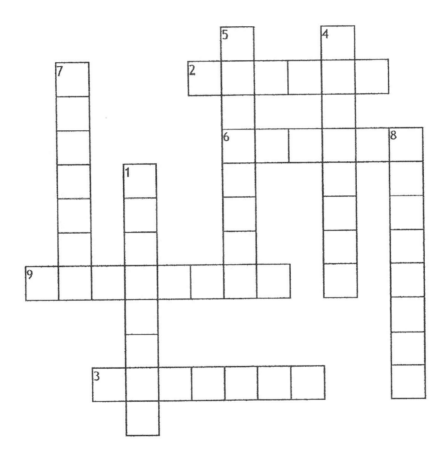

Across

2. What is Cisatracurium trade name?
3. What is Doxacurium trade name?
6. What is Pipecuronium trade name?
9. What is succinylcholine Trade name?

Down

1. What is Atracurium trade name?
4. What is Metocurine trade name?
5. What is Mivacurium trade name?
7. What is Rocuronium trade name?
8. What is Vecuronium trade name?

ADRENERGIC BLOCKERS (SYMPATHOLYTICS) MEDICATIONS

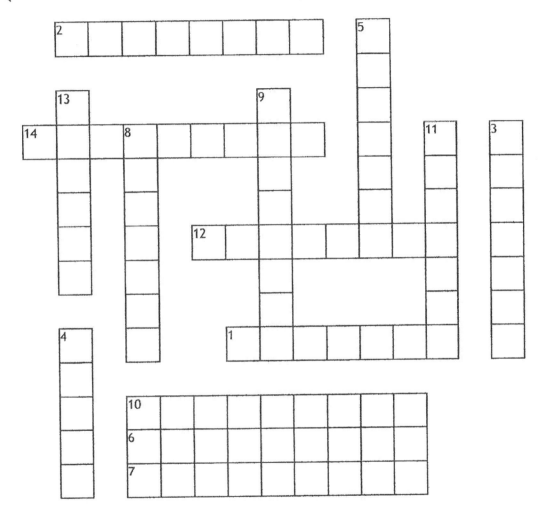

Across
1. What is Acebutolol trade name?
2. What is Atenolol trade name?
6. What is Esmolol trade name?
7. What is Metoprolol trade name?
10. What is Prazosin trade name?
12. What is Sotalol trade name?
14. What is timolol trade name?

Down
3. What is Carteolol trade name?
4. What is Carvedilol trade name?
5. What is Doxazosin trade name?
8. What is Nadolol trade name?
9. What is Phentolamine trade name?
11. What is Propranolol trade name?
13. What is Tamsulosin trade name?

GABA ACTION ANTISEIZURE MEDICATIONS I

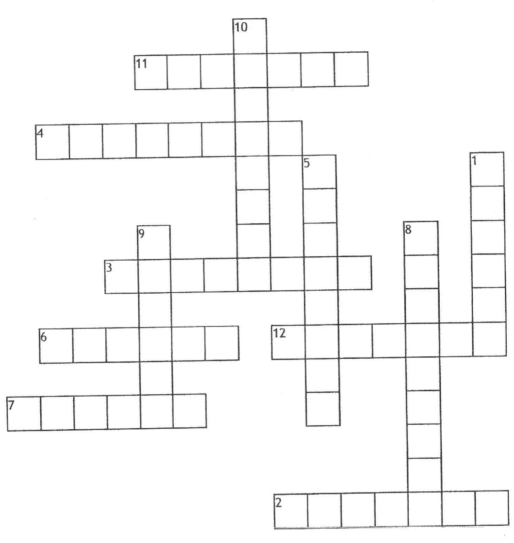

Across

2. What is phenobarbital trade name?
3. What is primidone trade name?
4. What is clonazepam trade name?
6. What is diazepam trade name?
7. What is lorazepam trade name?
11. What is topiramate trade name?
12. What is mephobarbital trade name?

Down

1. What is amobarbital trade name?
5. What is clorazepate dipotassium trade name?
8. What is gabapentin trade name?
9. What is pregabalin trade name?
10. What is tiagabine trade name?

GABA ACTION ANTISEIZURE MEDICATIONS II

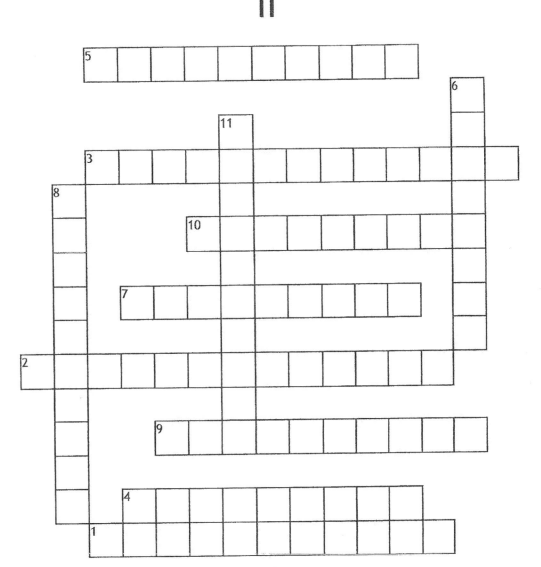

Across
1. What is Amytal generic name?
2. What is Mebaral generic name?
3. What is luminal generic name?
4. What is Mysoline generic name?
5. What is Klonopin generic name?
7. What is Ativan generic name?
9. What is Lyrica generic name?
10. What is Gabitril generic name?

Down
6. What is Valium generic name?
8. What is Neurontin generic name?
11. What is Topamax generic name?

MEDICATION ANTIDOTES

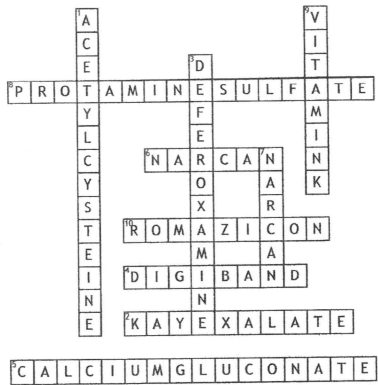

Across

2. What is Potassium's antidote?
4. What is digoxin antidote?
5. What is Magnesium Sulfate antidote?
6. What are Opiods antidote?
8. What is Heparin's antidote?
10. What is Benzodiazepines antidote?

Down

1. What is tylenol's antidote?
3. What is Iron's antidote?
7. What are Narcotics antidote?
9. What is Coumadin's antidote?

ATTENTION DEFICIT-HYPERACTIVITY DISORDER CNS STIMULANTS & NONSTIMULANTS MEDICATIONS

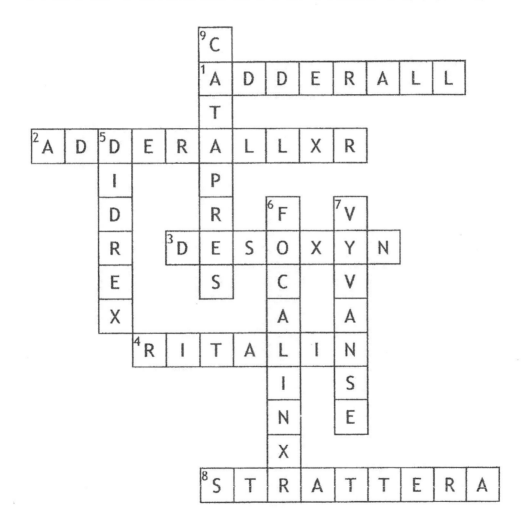

Across

1. What is d- & l-Amphetamine racemic mixture trade name?

2. What is Dextroamphetamine mixture trade name?

3. What is Methamphetamine trade name?

4. What is Methylphenidate trade name?

8. What is Atomoxetine trade name?

Down

5. What is Benzphetamine trade name?

6. What is Dexmethylphenidate trade name?

7. What is Lisdexamfetamine trade name?

9. What is Clonidine trade name?

SELECTIVE SEROTONIN REUPTAKE INHIBITORS (SSRIs) & SEROTONIN-NOREPINEPHRINE REUPTAKE INHIBITORS (SNRIs)

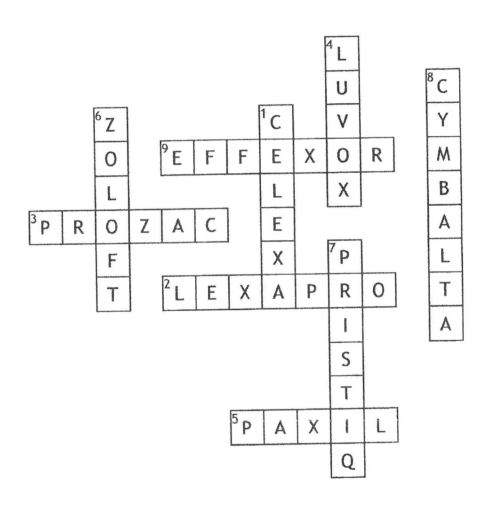

Across

2. What is Escitalopram Oxalate trade name?
3. What is Fluoxetine trade name?
5. What is Paroxetine trade name?
9. What is Venlafaxine trade name?

Down

1. What is Citalopram trade name?
4. What is Fluvoxamine trade name?
6. What is Sertraline trade name?
7. What is Desvenlafaxine trade name?
8. What is Duloxetine trade name?

ANTICONVULSANT MEDICATIONS

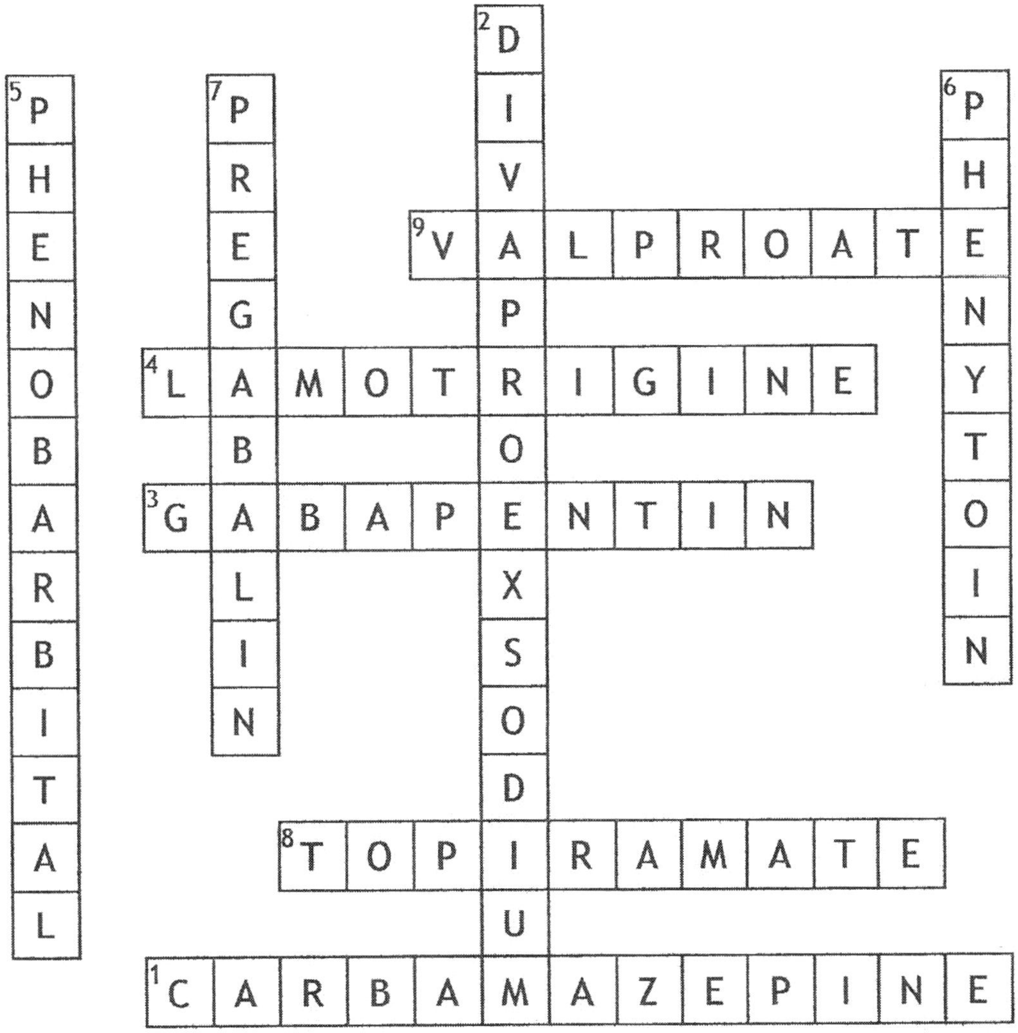
2 DIVALPROEX SODIUM
5 PHENOBARBITAL
7 PREGABALIN
6 PHENYTOIN
9 VALPROATE
4 LAMOTRIGINE
3 GABAPENTIN
8 TOPIRAMATE
1 CARBAMAZEPINE

Across

1. What is Tegretol generic name?
3. What is Neurontin generic name?
4. What is Lamictal generic name?
8. What is Topamax generic name?
9. What is Depacon generic name?

Down

2. What is Depakote generic name?
5. What is luminal generic name?
6. What is Dilantin generic name?
7. What is Lyrica generic name?

ANTIPSYCHOTIC MEDICATIONS

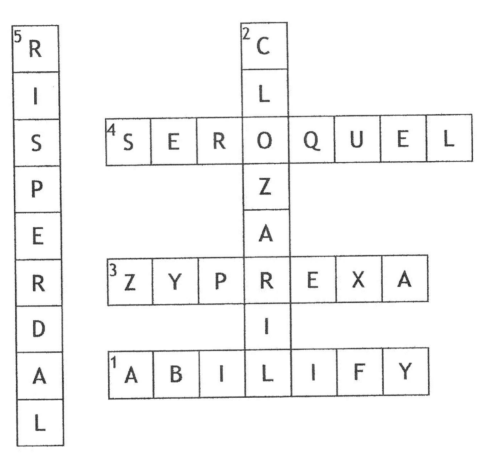

Across

1. What is Aripiprazole trade name?
3. What is Olanzepine trade name?
4. What is Quetiapine Fumarate trade name?

Down

2. What s Clozapine trade name?
5. What is Risperidone trade name?

PARKINSON'S ANTICHOLINERGIC MEDS

```
                          ¹B
      ²A                   E                ³C
      K         ⁴A         N                 O
      I          R         A                 G
      N          T         D                 E
⁵K  E   M   A   D   R   I   N
      T          N         Y                 T
      O          E         L                 I
      N                                      N
```

Across

5. What is Procyclidine trade name?

Down

1. What is Diphenhydramine trade name?
2. What is Biperiden trade name?
3. What is Benzotropine trade name?
4. What is Trihexyphenidyl trade name?

ALZHEIMER'S ACETYLCHOLINESTERASE INHIBITORS MEDICATIONS

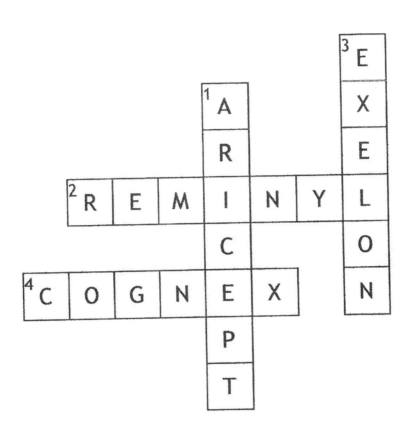

Across
2. What is Galantamine trade name?
4. What is Tacrine trade name?

Down
1. What is Donepezil trade name?
3. What is Rivastigmine Tartrate trade name?

MULTIPLE SCLEROSIS MEDICATIONS

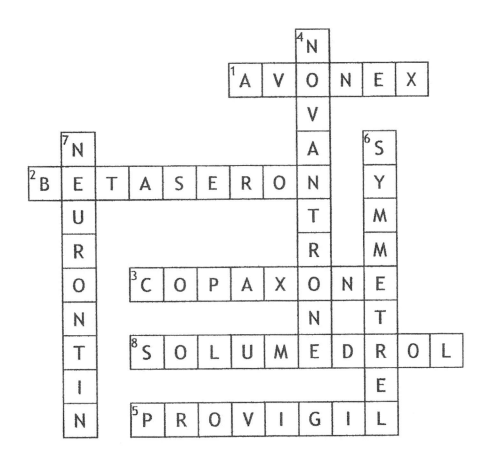

Across

1. What is Interferon beta-1 a trade name?
2. What is Interferon beta-1 b trade name?
3. What is Glatiramer Acetate trade name?
5. What is Modafinil trade name?
8. What is Methylprednisolone trade name?

Down

4. What is Mitoxantrone trade name?
6. What s Amantadine trade name?
7. What is Gabapentin trade name?

NONPHENOTHIAZINES CONVENTIONAL ANTIPSYCHOTICS MEDICATIONS

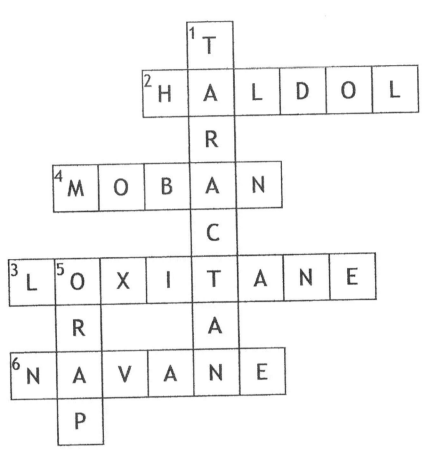

Across
2. What is Haloperidol trade name?
3. What is Loxapine Succinate trade name?
4. What is Molindone HCL trade name?
6. What is Thiothixene HCL trade name?

Down
1. What is Chlorprothixene trade name?
5. What is Pimozide trade name?

ANTISPASMATIC MEDICATIONS

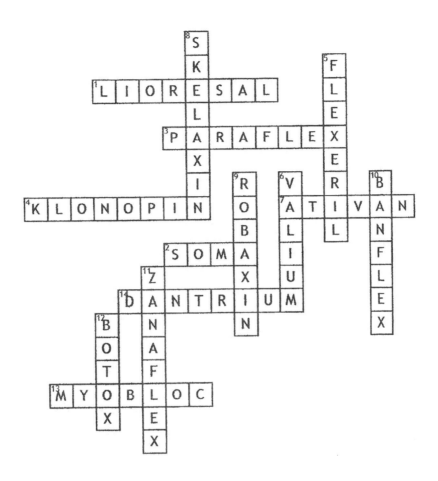

Across

1. What is Baclofen trade name?
2. What is Carisoprodol trade name?
3. What is Chlorzoxazone trade name?
4. What is Clonazepam trade name?
7. What is Lorazepam trade name?
13. What is Botulinum toxin type B trade name?
14. What is Dantrolene Sodium trade name?

Down

5. What is Cyclobenzaprine trade name?
6. What is Diazepam trade name?
8. What is Metaxalone trade name?
9. What is Methocarbamol trade name?
10. What is Orphenadrine Citrate trade name?
11. What is Tizanidine trade name?
12. What is Botulinum toxin type A trade name?

SYMPATHOMIMETICS MEDICATIONS

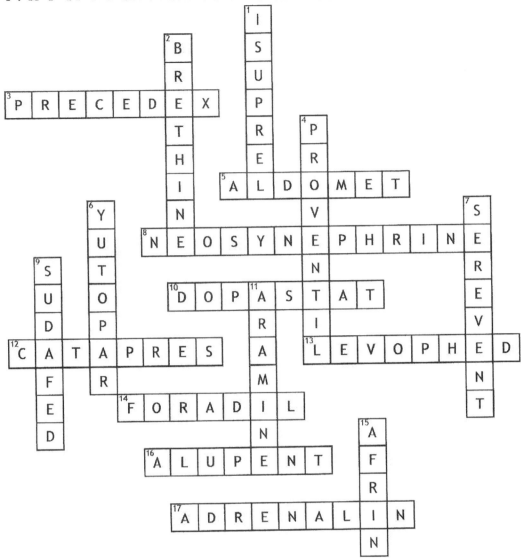

Across
3. What is Dexmedetomidine HCL trade name?
5. What is methyldopa trade name?
8. What is Phenylephrine trade name?
10. What is Dobutamine trade name?
12. What is Clonidine trade name?
13. What is norepinephrine trade name?
14. What is Formoterol trade name?
16. What is Metaproterenol trade name?
17. What is Ephinephrine trade name?

Down
1. What is Isoproterenol trade name?
2. What is Terbutaline trade name?
4. What is Albuterol trade name?
6. What is Ritodrine trade name?
7. What is Salmeterol trade name?
9. What is Pseudophedrine trade name?
11. What is Metaraminol trade name?
15. What is Oxymetazoline trade name?

PARASYMPATHOMIMETICS MEDICATIONS

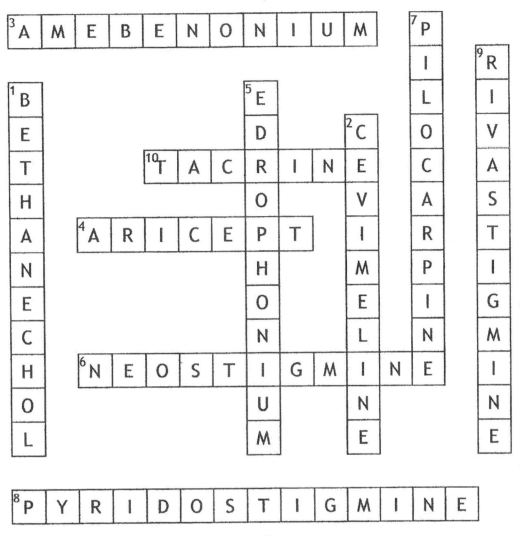

Across

3. What is Mytelase generic name?
4. What is Donepezil generic name?
6. What is Prostigmin generic name?
8. What is Mestinon generic name?
10. What is Cognex generic name?

Down

1. What is Urecholine generic name?
2. What is Evoxac generic name?
5. What is Tensilon generic name?
7. What is Isopto Carpine generic name?
9. What is Exelon generic name?

PARASYMPATHOMIMETIC MEDICATIONS II

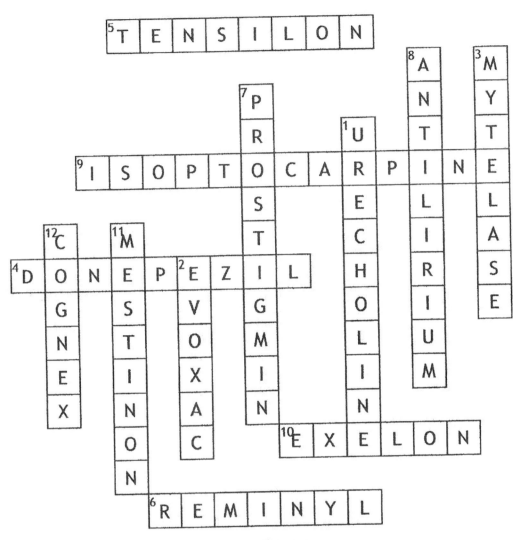

Across
4. What is the trade name for Aricept?
5. What is the trade name for Edrophonium?
6. What is the trade name for Galantamine Hydrobromide
9. What is the trade name for Pilocarpine?
10. What is the trade name for Rivastigmine?

Down
1. What is the trade name for Bethanechol?
2. What is the trade name for Cevimeline HCL
3. What is the trade name for Amebenonium CHL?
7. What is the trade name for Neostigmine?
8. What is the trade name for Physostigmine?
11. What is the trade name for Pyridostigmine?
12. What is the trade name for Tacrine?

NUEROMUSCULAR BLOCKING MEDICATIONS

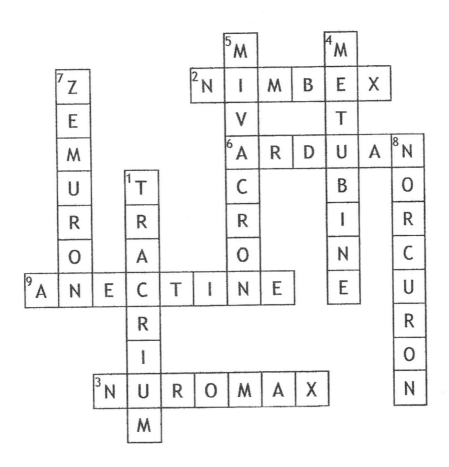

Across

2. What is Cisatracurium trade name?
3. What is Doxacurium trade name?
6. What is Pipecuronium trade name?
9. What is succinylcholine Trade name?

Down

1. What is Atracurium trade name?
4. What is Metocurine trade name?
5. What is Mivacurium trade name?
7. What is Rocuronium trade name?
8. What is Vecuronium trade name?

ADRENERGIC BLOCKERS (SYMPATHOLYTICS) MEDICATIONS

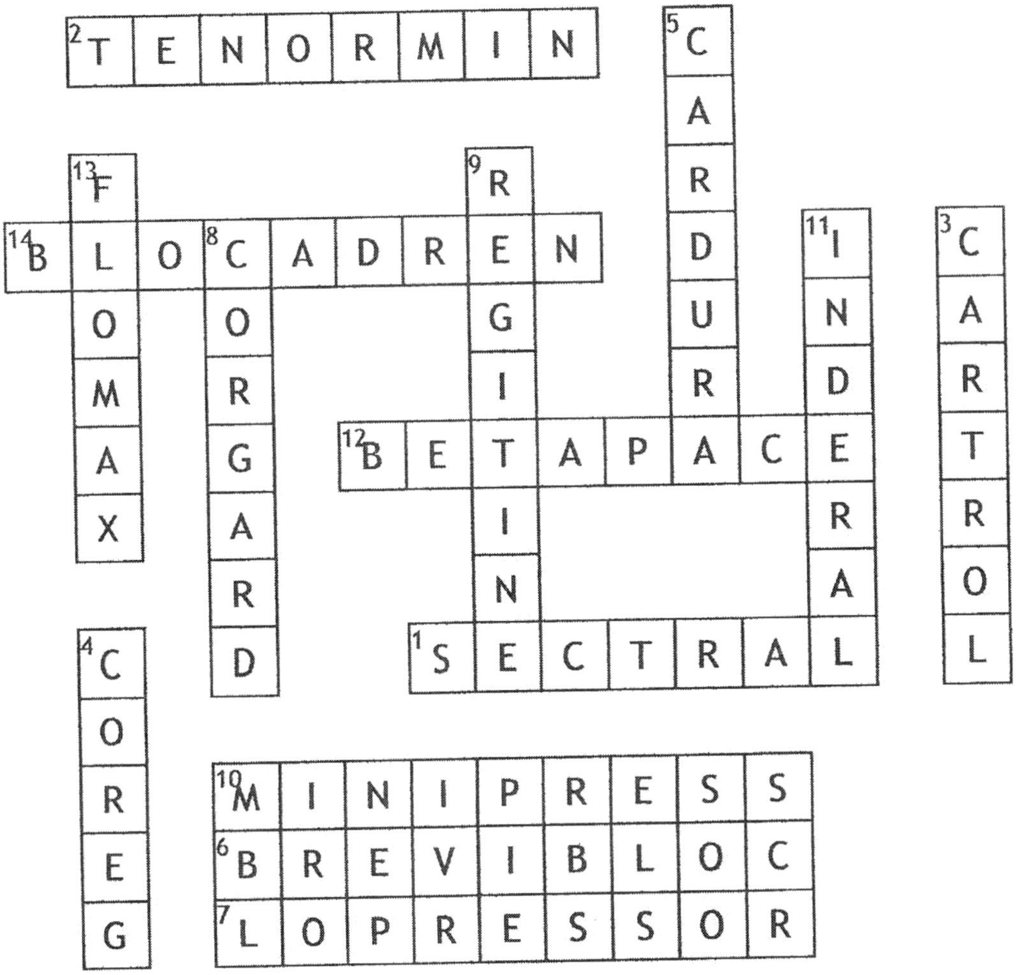

Crossword grid answers:

- 2 Across: TENORMIN
- 14 Across: BLOCADREN
- 12 Across: BETAPACE
- 1 Across: SECTRAL
- 10 Across: MINIPRESS
- 6 Across: BREVIBLOC
- 7 Across: LOPRESSOR
- 13 Down: FLOMAX
- 8 Down: CORGARD
- 9 Down: REGITINE
- 5 Down: CARDURA
- 11 Down: INDERAL
- 3 Down: CARTROL
- 4 Down: COREG

Across

1. What is Acebutolol trade name?
2. What is Atenolol trade name?
6. What is Esmolol trade name?
7. What is Metoprolol trade name?
10. What is Prazosin trade name?
12. What is Sotalol trade name?
14. What is timolol trade name?

Down

3. What is Carteolol trade name?
4. What is Carvedilol trade name?
5. What is Doxazosin trade name?
8. What is Nadolol trade name?
9. What is Phentolamine trade name?
11. What is Propranolol trade name?
13. What is Tamsulosin trade name?

GABA ACTION ANTISEIZURE MEDICATIONS I

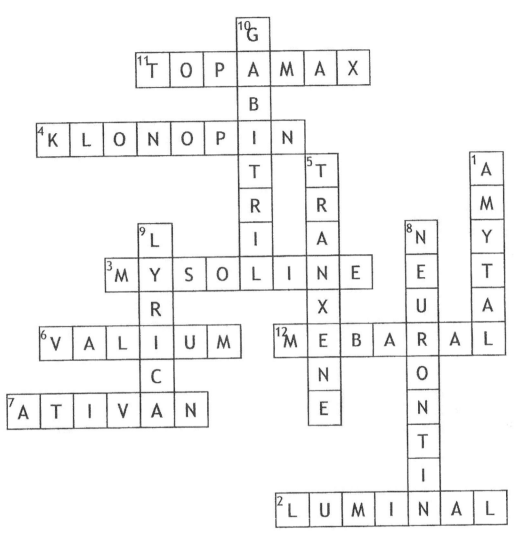

Across

2. What is phenobarbital trade name?
3. What is primidone trade name?
4. What is clonazepam trade name?
6. What is diazepam trade name?
7. What is lorazepam trade name?
11. What is topiramate trade name?
12. What is mephobarbital trade name?

Down

1. What is amobarbital trade name?
5. What is clorazepate dipotassium trade name?
8. What is gabapentin trade name?
9. What is pregabalin trade name?
10. What is tiagabine trade name?

GABA ACTION ANTISEIZURE MEDICATIONS II

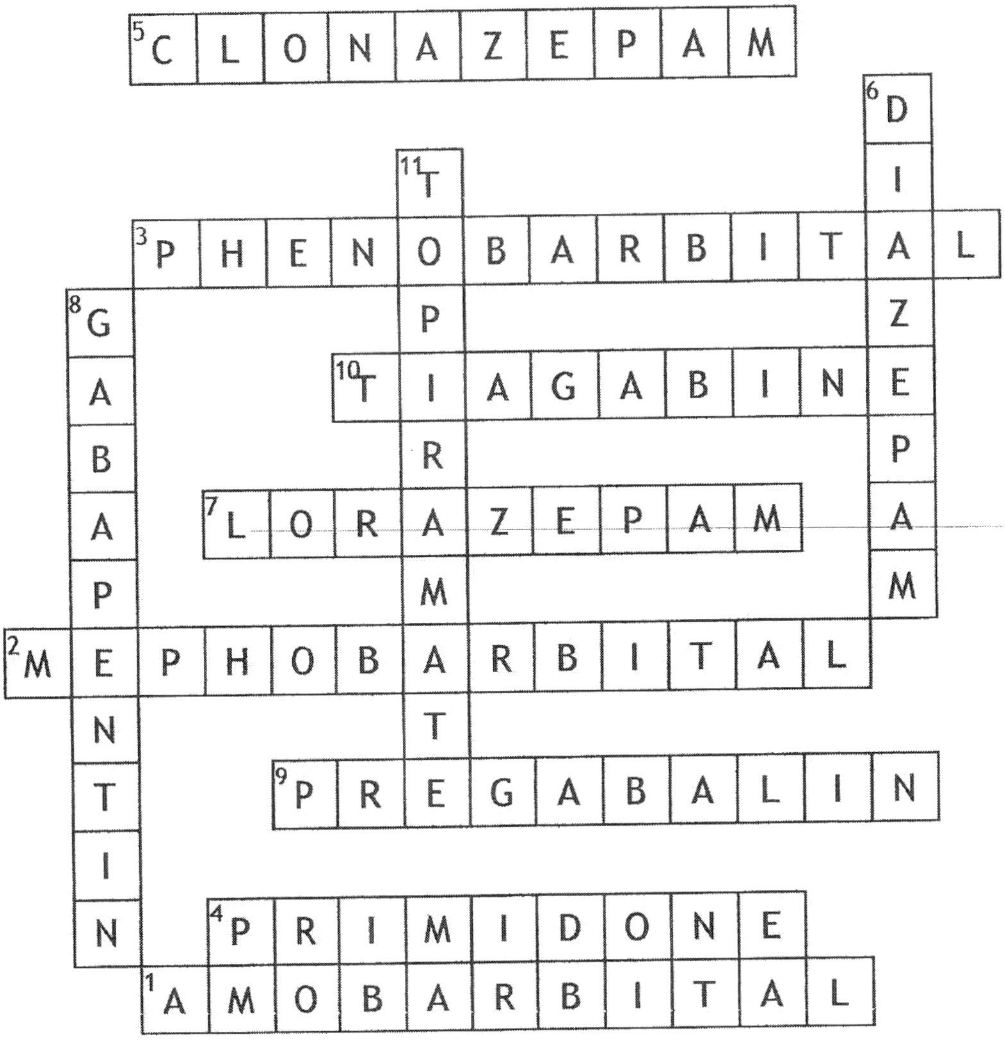
5 CLONAZEPAM
6 DIAZEPAM
11 TOPIRAMATE
3 PHENOBARBITAL
8 GABAPENTIN
10 TIAGABINE
7 LORAZEPAM
2 MEPHOBARBITAL
9 PREGABALIN
4 PRIMIDONE
1 AMOBARBITAL

Across

1. What is Amytal generic name?
2. What is Mebaral generic name?
3. What is luminal generic name?
4. What is Mysoline generic name?
5. What is Klonopin generic name?
7. What is Ativan generic name?
9. What is Lyrica generic name?
10. What is Gabitril generic name?

Down

6. What is Valium generic name?
8. What is Neurontin generic name?
11. What is Topamax generic name?

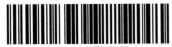
Made in the USA
San Bernardino, CA
16 July 2019